I0758987

THE INTERMITTENT DIET

The complete guide with delicious recipes to easily follow the 16:8 regime of the intermittent diet and lose weight fast

16 hours fasted

Paul Fung

THE INTERMITTENT DIET 16:8

The complete guide with delicious recipes to easily follow the 16: 8 regime of the intermittent diet and lose weight fast

EDITED BY PAUL FUNG

Legal notes

The strategies reported in this manual are the result of years of studies, therefore the achievement of the same results is not guaranteed. The author reserves the right to update or modify the content based on new conditions. The author of this book does not dispense medical advice or prescribe the use of any techniques, advice, or suggestions as a form of treatment for physical, emotional, or medical problems without the advice of a physician. The author's intent is based on personal experience and has the sole purpose of offering general information in the pursuit of greater well-being. In the event that you use any of the information contained in this book, the author assumes no responsibility for your actions.

TABLE OF CONTENTS

INTRODUCTION

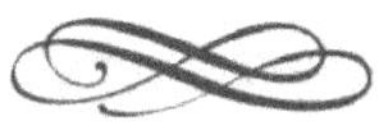

1. Healthy and tasty

The main difference between a common diet and a meal plan is that the former is temporary while the latter is a lifestyle.

If you say "From Monday to start" this is a diet, it is usually restrictive, it resembles a punishment and assumes that there are certain types of prohibited foods. A diet sounds like this: "I can't eat cookies anymore, I'm on a diet" or "Pizza? No thanks. I'm on a diet." Or "Oh ... I really want ice cream but I'm on a diet and it's so hard to resist .. Ok, ok only this time and then I won't go wrong anymore ".

This module usually leads to feelings of guilt and consequently to eating even more. It's a diet!

If you say "I would like to feel better, feel healthier and more vital", then you are looking for a lifestyle change.

A lifestyle change sounds like this: "Well, I had a healthy breakfast, lunch was balanced, I gave my body a lot of nutrients. I can eat a cookie and it won't make much difference. Especially since I'm planning on having a light dinner ".

This usually helps you stick to a healthy eating plan, feel better, lose weight, and keep fit.

So, as you can deduce, a healthy eating plan doesn't mean you have to give up on taste or your favorite foods. It simply means balance and moderation.

Healthy food is not necessarily tasteless. The key is to give your body the nutrients it needs to stay healthy and give you energy. If you choose your favorite healthy foods, then you can go looking for different recipes and prepare those foods in many ways.

If your diet is balanced and healthy overall, you can give yourself an extra, from time to time. Even among these extras you can choose the higher quality ones. Let's take some examples.

Let's say you really like ice cream. Instead of buying packaged, low-quality, chemical-filled ice cream, you can choose artisanal ice cream made with genuine ingredients. The same goes for cookies, pizza or bread.

The real problem is those foods that are not even "real foods" and could be defined as "artificial". These include industrially manufactured products and beverages that don't even exist in nature. You can recognize them by the color (they are usually very colorful such as sugar-coated chocolate candies) and by the list of ingredients on the package (very long with names that are difficult to pronounce or even to read).

When I say "the real problem", what I mean is that your body does not recognize those foods, does not know what to do with them and therefore they pollute your body, create imbalances and in the long run they can generate diseases.

Now that we have clarified the difference between a food plan and a diet, that we have recognized that healthy can be tasty, we can say that although it is called the "Intermittent Fasting Diet", it is not a diet in the most common way that the word is used. . This regimen goes beyond the concept of diet and is a lifestyle change.

Above all, it is referred to as a diet when it comes to the various methods in which it can be followed. More on later in this guide.

2. The body needs nutrients

Just because a meal plan is a lifestyle change, and not a diet, that doesn't mean calories don't matter. If you follow a healthy eating plan, you still need to be aware of the calories you consume and the calories you burn if you want to lose weight.

It is a simple mathematical calculation. It is not possible to lose weight if your calorie intake is higher than the calories burned.

That said, it is important to note that your body needs nutrients and if you give it enough nutrients it will reward you with a lot of energy and won't continue to feel the constant desire to eat.

If you consider the so-called "comfort food" something to be given occasionally and not the norm, you will automatically reduce your calorie intake.

By following a healthy eating plan, instead of a temporary diet, you will focus on nutrient-rich foods and minimize calories from prepackaged high-carb and junk foods.

The solution to a healthier lifestyle is to give your body enough nutrients so it can function at its best.

Think of it like this, in order to carry out all daily activities, the body needs fuel and nutritious food is that fuel. Eating is about energizing your body, not just filling your stomach. In fact, you may even be full while your body starves (needs nutrients).

Nutritious foods for the body are those that belong to various groups of macronutrients such as carbohydrates and healthy fats, proteins, fibers, vitamins and minerals. The simpler the foods, the better. We will talk about specific foods in more detail later.

3. Keep your body strong

Obesity is a huge phenomenon, especially in Western countries, and is still on the rise to the point that it is starting to spread even in the East where it has never been before.

The problem of overweight and obesity goes beyond physical appearance. It is a serious problem that can lead to illness and in extreme cases even death.

What Causes Obesity? One could say: overeating. But overeating is an addiction, and an addiction is usually a cover for something deeper. It is usually an emotional problem. They are called "comfort food" for a reason.

Comfort foods are addictive if you overdo it. But, as we said before, some foods are artificial, produced industrially and not by nature. These processed foods are not recognized by the body and cause great imbalances.

All of these foods raise blood sugar levels and this in turn leads to fat accumulation and insensitivity to insulin.

It could also be argued that healthy options are much more expensive, but is that really true in the long run? Being healthy doesn't cost much in the way of medications and doctor visits. It actually costs nothing. Being sick, on the other hand, can be extremely expensive. And that's one thing. The other thing is that I always suggest choosing quality over quantity.

You don't have to eat four scoops of ice cream; you can eat two of superior quality. You don't have to eat steak every day, it's best to eat quality meat two or three times a week.

The same concept applies to all types of food.

By feeding your body with healthy and nutritious foods, avoiding simple carbohydrates (which are basically sugar in all its many forms), unhealthy - saturated - fats and "fake" foods (that is, all those that are defined as "empty calories" because contain no nutritional value), you are on the right path to amazing results.

Another reason that causes excess weight and in extreme cases obesity is the type of lifestyle you lead. Staying active keeps the body strong and alive. A sedentary lifestyle weakens the body. Everything is in the habits. But the good news is, you can break a habit. It takes dedication, perseverance, some time and practice.

A step at a time. You can go for a walk instead of watching another episode of your favorite show on TV. You can eat an apple instead of drinking sugar-filled bottled apple juice. All of these things matter. The transformation is the result of many small steps taken every day, it is not a leap you make overnight.

Working out helps you choose healthier foods. This is because - after exercise - you feel more energized, more gritty and cleaner but also because you don't want to ruin all the hard work you did by eating badly.

That said, it is now clear that the combination of leading an active lifestyle and selecting the right foods are the two factors working together to keep the body strong.

4. Keep the goal in mind

At first, your body will rebel against changes in your eating style. You can help yourself by imagining that you are dealing with a child and changing a few rules. The baby will cry a lot and moan at first but if you stay calm and patient, and don't give up, after a while the baby will learn and accept the new rules. The same goes for your body. Treat it with patience but be firm in your decision and keep your goal in mind.

Since adapting to a new diet is not the easiest thing to do, the thing to do, before even starting, is to make a decision and stick to it.

To do this, it is essential that you have clear in mind why you are doing it: what is your motivation? The reasons are varied and one is no longer valid on the other. It could be to look good in your skinny jeans or have the energy to play with your kids or dog, stay healthy and vital, get ready for a wedding or romantic vacation, to boost self-esteem etc. .

Whatever it is, be sure to keep the goal in mind. This will especially help you in times of hunger and when you feel sad or discouraged.

It may also be helpful to have a vision board with inspiring images and quotes to keep you motivated about your weight loss and health goals.

You may want to keep a list of the benefits of intermittent fasting (we'll explore them later), exercise, and eat nutritious foods with you to remind yourself of your motives.

If you stick to the new habits, it will get easier as you go.

PART I
OVERVIEW OF INTERMITTENT FASTING

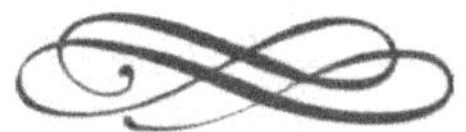

1. Intermittent Fasting: The Basics

Intermittent fasting is a meal plan that requires you to go through phases   you can eat and phases you can't eat. Intermittent fasting, although only recently being adopted for weight and health benefits, has been around for many, many years. It is a food model widely used not only by athletes but by all types of people including men, women, teenagers etc.

Most people fast daily without even realizing it. Think about the concept of breakfast… Breakfast breaks the fast of the night.

Since intermittent fasting is considered a method of cleansing and detoxifying the body, it is an option many people choose to improve their overall health and can also help those who are looking to get fit and lose weight.

The intermittent fasting diet is sometimes called the "famine diet". It's not a new trend, it's actually been around for quite some time. The reason it has spread is that it has proven effective for a great many people.

Fasting has existed in one form or another since the beginning of humanity. Recently, it has spread among athletes, fitness enthusiasts and people who need to follow a diet. More and more people are fasting to get rid of toxins, to improve their health and to lose excess fat.

Some appreciate its practicality and simplicity. Others are confused by the variety of different regimens that involve the intermittent diet.

There are some common questions when it comes to diets. Including:

- What can you eat on fasting days?
- What is allowed and what is forbidden?
- Do you need to track calories?
- Should I include all macronutrients or should I exclude carbohydrates?
- Should I be careful with portions or can I eat as much as I think I need?
- Can I avoid exercising since I am on a diet?

In this Guide, we will answer the questions above and address other diet-related topics, as well as trying to eliminate any doubts and confusion about the intermittent fasting diet.

2. Intermittent fasting: various formulas

(Brief explanation of the methods of fasting)

There are different regimes within the intermittent fasting diet. The main difference is the various stages you eat and the stages you fast.

There is more than one way to follow the fasting regime. In reality, there are many types of protocol to choose from. To select the right one for you, you need to have a brief overview of the different methods and then decide according to your needs, program and other factors.

Intermittent fasting mainly changes the times you eat since the element that sets this program apart from any other diet is "when" (when to eat and when to fast).

16: 8

One of the simplest methods to follow, and therefore also the most popular, is 16: 8. Easier because it is the one where you actually fast for a shorter period of time during your waking hours.

What happens is that you fast for 16 hours and you can eat your meals during the remaining 8 hours. The fact is, most of the fasting phase happens during sleep, which, as you can infer, makes it easier to stick to the regimen.

Let's say you enjoy dining with your family, so you don't want to give up on this meal, as a result you may want to start your 16 hours of fasting from after dinner until the next day.

Also be sure to keep in mind what are the times of the day when you tend to be really hungry and plan accordingly.

Eat-fast-Eat

Another method is called Eat-Stop-Eat. This is a bit more difficult because it requires you to stand 24 hours straight without eating. It's a full day!

If you choose this method, you may want to do it once or twice a week. If you've never been on a diet, or are just starting out, you might want to try a full day of fasting per week.

Remember not to drink the calories! There must be no calorie intake during the 24-hour period, so plain water is the best choice, although you can also have tea or coffee as long as you don't add sugar, milk or cream.

It goes without saying that for the rest of the week it is best to keep the body healthy and vital by making wise food choices. Choose nutritious and delicious foods, foods that make you feel good and clean.

To follow this protocol, for example, you can start in the morning and fast until the next day, or you can start around noon. And this is what most people prefer to do.

The method of the warrior

This regime is called "The Warrior" because you have to be a warrior to survive a longer period of fasting. It is one of the strictest methods of intermittent fasting. In fact, the reason it is called the warrior method is that it comes from a Paleo Diet concept of eating like our ancestors who had to go out to hunt and forage for food and could only eat when food was available, when they were able to find or procure it.

To follow this protocol, you eat a large meal and then fast for the next 24 hours.

Another feature of the warrior method is that you have to stick to the cavemen's eating habits when eating! A bit like Paleo but not really ... Just common sense ... Ask yourself: what would an ancestor eat? Meat, fish, fruit, vegetables ... the simplest things, the basic foods for survival, nothing special and elaborate.

Be aware of the quality of the foods you choose. When buying meat, for example, opt for that which comes from naturally fed animals, choose free-range eggs and poultry. This should be the case not only if you are following the warrior method, but also if you are aiming for a healthier lifestyle.

If possible, buy local, fresh and seasonal products. If you make a habit of buying these types of products, you will have the opportunity to enjoy foods, especially meat, free of hormones and other chemicals. The benefits to your overall health will be nothing short of amazing.

Fasting every other day

Another way to follow the intermittent fasting diet is alternate day fasting. To do this, fast every other day. You can experiment and for example choose the 16: 8 method every other day or maybe follow a full 24 hours of fasting every other day.

Choose what works best for you, based on your schedule and the messages you get from your body. This means that you have to pay attention to how you feel!

Some people choose to only include water (coffee or tea) when fasting, others include up to 500 calories.

5: 2

The 5: 2 works like this: you eat for 5 days and fast the other 2 of the week. Again, that doesn't mean you can eat pasta, bread and pizza for 5 days in a row and then nothing for two days. Keep a clean and fresh diet, you can still eat a pizza every now and then, indeed you can still have all your favorite foods if you consume them in moderation and if they are of good quality, made with fresh and genuine ingredients.

While the general idea behind intermittent fasting remains the same, there are many variations of intermittent fasting that serve as perfect diet plans for different people depending on their personal needs, preferences and goals.

Before we discuss the different most common types of intermittent fasting diets, there are a few things you need to keep in mind. When considering adopting any type of intermittent fasting diet, remember that different methods will produce different results. While they will all provide various benefits in their own way, they will work differently for different people.

When deciding to choose the intermittent fasting diet, don't force yourself into a certain regimen. If you find that one method is too difficult, it may not be the right option for you. For a diet to work, it is essential that you have an open mind and a positive approach.

If you don't want the benefits of the diet to be short-lived, always choose a diet plan that fits your lifestyle so you can stick to it for the long term. This will make it easier for you to achieve your goals.

3. Intermittent fasting: various formulas

In the context of intermittent fasting, alternating phases in which you eat and phases in which you fast. Fasting is considered a period of time in which you give your body a kind of "rest" and the chance to purify itself. It's like a detox. Not eating allows the body to regenerate and use the nutrients it has previously received.

Fasting also helps regulate and stabilize insulin (sugar) levels in the blood. This is a good thing because as a result you will no longer feel those sudden and unstoppable pangs of hunger.

During the fasting period the body burns fat. The extra caloric intake turns into fat which is stored in the body as "supply". Fasting causes the body to use that "supply" and burn it.

The body tends to burn immediately available energy (the one that comes from the food you just ate). Unless necessary, it does not burn the "reserve".

As we said, the intermittent fasting feeding schedule consists of two phases: feeding period and fasting period, these are also referred to as windows.

Since certain foods are harder to resist when hungry, make sure you always have healthy food available during the eating window.

As you continue with your healthy eating plan, constant hunger will be reduced and the sugar dips that are so common when you are not aware of your eating habits will be reduced.

So the idea of intermittent fasting is to follow these healthy guidelines during the eating window and allow the body to clean up while fasting.

The intermittent fasting program can help you lose weight if you are aware of some misperceptions.

For example, just because you are fasting for a certain period of time does not mean that you can eat as much as you want during the eating phase.

Also, if you want to lose weight and feel healthier, you need to choose a type of physical activity that you enjoy. It doesn't have to be extreme, but you should work out at least 20 minutes almost every day.

There are so many activities to choose from and you can even watch workout videos on YouTube and follow them in the comfort of your own home if you don't have time to hit the gym. Or you could run, ride a bike, go for a swim, do aerobics or pilates, play tennis. The options are endless.

If you are following the intermittent fasting diet but are not losing weight, it may be that you are drinking your calories without realizing it, without counting them. Drinks (if caloric) matter as much as food. Many people drink their calories through sugar-dense carbonated sodas that are full of chemicals.

If you choose foods high in sugar and carbohydrates during the eating window such as croissants for breakfast, cake and cookies in the afternoon, and pizza for dinner, it doesn't matter if you fast, you won't lose weight or feel better.

Also, if this is the type of food you eat regularly, it will be much more difficult for you to fast because food that is high in carbohydrates, simple carbohydrates - like baked goods - make you want to eat more and more.

As with all things in life, it takes some time to adjust to new habits. So at first you may even feel worse than before and feel like you are always hungry. This is because the body is getting rid of all toxins and, unless you decide to give up, you will gradually adapt.

Before starting your fast, try to allow longer periods of time between meals, as well as cutting down on simple carbohydrates and sugars, and increasing protein and fiber (more fruits and vegetables). Start doing this for about 3 weeks before starting the new program.

4. Intermittent fasting: advantages and disadvantages

Many people find it difficult not to think about food while fasting. This is especially true if you treat it as some kind of punishment and count the hours before the fasting window is over.

Keep in mind that fasting is not about avoiding food, but about giving your body a break.

I suggest that you treat fasting as a rejuvenating time for yourself and your body. Taking a more positive approach will make it easier to follow.

Hunger can cause anger!

Some people become very irritable when they are hungry. And this is a disadvantage. The body likes routines and if you don't give it enough food at the appointed time you may notice that even a trivial matter can cause anger or irritation.

You could use this opportunity as a practice to become more aware of your feelings and their cause. Start paying more attention to your state of mind. After a while, as we have already mentioned, the body adjusts to the new program. Also, in these cases, listening to music and walking outdoors really helps a lot.

Initially, fasting can also cause headaches and fatigue. These are usually the symptoms of hypoglycemia, which is essentially a lack of sugar in the bloodstream.

This condition is especially likely to happen to people who have developed some kind of addiction to certain foods that are full of fat and sugar. Your body will need time to adjust to dips in energy and although you may be tempted to snack because you feel cravings, you recognize that it is an addiction - a sugar addiction - so if you give up, if you don't break the habit, you stay employeed.

Since fasting lowers blood sugar, intermittent fasting is not recommended for those with low blood sugar or those diagnosed with diabetes. Therefore, you should consult with your doctor before deciding to incorporate intermittent fasting into your lifestyle.

One of the biggest benefits of the intermittent fasting diet is its simplicity. Once you know the basics of healthy eating, such as the major nutrient groups (protein, fiber, healthy fats, vitamins and minerals, and different types of carbohydrates) and how different foods affect the body, you simply need to plan and keep the initial enthusiasm high.

Thanks to intermittent fasting, you are likely to learn to eat better overall.

When it comes to losing weight, calorie counting obviously matters. Research has shown that, on average, a group of people who support the intermittent fasting diet consumes at least 350 fewer calories per day than the same group that doesn't follow the same meal plan. When you only have a limited window of time in which to eat, the result is that you don't eat as much food as usual. This automatically limits your total calorie intake, leading to weight loss.

Based on various factors, including body mass index, age, gender and lifestyle, find out how many calories you need to maintain the weight you want and maintain that calorie level.

Other benefits of this regimen include better cardiovascular function, a stronger immune system, and a decrease in blood pressure.

When the intermittent fasting diet is followed correctly, it regulates appetite and keeps hunger at bay.

Intermittent fasting is not considered a good idea for everyone. For example, it is not a suitable regimen for those people who are underweight.

Also, intermittent fasting is NOT indicated if ...

You have tried it and you continue to feel bad even after a short adjustment period.

Some people have low blood sugar and other conditions that may not allow them to fast. If you feel dizzy, weak, or just plain sick, break your fast and eat something nutritious.

Listen to your body and proceed accordingly. It is normal to experience fatigue and headaches at first, but these symptoms should disappear in a short time.

Intermittent fasting is probably not suitable for people with particular health conditions. It is always important to consult your doctor before starting a diet or training program.

If you have diabetes, do not start this diet unless you get the consent of your doctor. This type of plan has an impact on your blood sugar and, in the event of an imbalance due to diabetes, it could be harmful to your health. Regardless of whether you have a health condition or not, always consult your doctor first. This is essential to be able to proceed safely.

5. Intermittent fasting: science and history (some research)

The origin of the intermittent fasting diet dates back to the way our ancestors ate. At the time, food wasn't around the corner. No refrigerator, no electricity, no fast food, no cars and no home deliveries. If you wanted to eat, you had to grow your own fruits and vegetables, you had to hunt or go fishing somewhere. The result is that the food was not only scarce (not available every day, and this is the idea behind fasting) but it was also very simple, unprocessed, unpackaged and without added chemicals.

Simply cooked, perhaps directly on the stove, perhaps with a little salt ... That's all.

On the days when you were able to get food from hunting, fishing or a good harvest, it was a real celebration. If, on the other hand, the resources were scarce and there was no food, you would have gone hungry. The only difference between this and the intermittent fasting diet is that you had no choice in the past.

Because of this way of eating and fasting, and because the food was very simple and genuine, our ancestors were not overweight. They knew nothing about obesity. Also, keep in mind that hunting, fishing and growing vegetables is considered the version of the gym activities of our ancestors.

Intermittent fasting has been the subject of extensive research. The results of these numerous studies on intermittent fasting have shown that it can have a positive effect on cognitive health as well. This means it can improve brain and memory health. As a result, you can reduce the risk of brain diseases such as dementia and Alzheimer's.

This food program improves insulin sensitivity, increases metabolism and keeps the heart healthy. Also, the body burns stored fat instead of sugar for more energy.

In addition to reducing hunger, improving mental focus, and lowering blood glucose levels, alternating between periods of fasting and eating can preserve muscle strength. Compared to other weight loss methods, intermittent dieting does not cause muscle tone loss. Most athletes who adopt intermittent fasting experience greater energy and strength, greater focus and better performance.

By reducing blood sugar and insulin levels, following the intermittent diet helps maintain constant energy throughout the day. It also lowers LDL cholesterol, which is the bad type, and increases HDL, which is the good type. This consequently helps reduce the risk of heart disease.

INTERMITTENT FASTING 16: 8

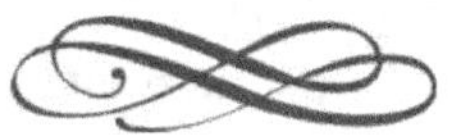

1. What is the 16: 8 method?

The 16: 8 method consists of a 16-hour fasting window and an 8-hour feeding window. If you have dinner at 7pm and have breakfast at 11am the next day, you have fasted for 16 hours.

But, let's go into more detail. If you have an 8-hour feeding window and a 16-hour fasting window, you will need to consume all the calories of the day during the 8 hours. In the example above, this would mean between 11.00 and 19.00.

For this reason, many believe that the 16: 8 method is the best solution for following the intermittent fasting diet. It is very close to what is considered "the norm" and therefore, easy enough to follow and stick to it without starving, feeling punished or experiencing fatigue and loss of energy.

I find that usually the simple things work best. If you have to start following complex patterns, strategies to avoid carbohydrates, charts, endless lists and strange ingredients to incorporate into your diet, it is much easier for you to decide to give up everything after a short period of time.

What you need, however, is motivation and self-discipline, and that comes naturally when you have a clear idea of why you are doing what you are doing. If you have a goal to achieve, you can tolerate some discomfort. If you have no purpose, no willpower will ever be enough.

2. 16: 8 method for beginners

If long periods of fasting scare you, if 24 hours seems like a long time to fast, you might choose to start by trying the 16-hour fast. This is considered one of the easiest because about half of the 16 hours are spent sleeping.

If you follow this type of intermittent fasting schedule, which is the 16: 8 method, you have an eight hour feeding window. The feeding period should ideally be around noon so your body doesn't process insulin when you sleep. However, as you begin, try different methods to gauge their impact on your routine and body. If it's causing you too much stress and discomfort, it's time to reevaluate your diet, take a deep breath, and try a different way.

Try to avoid stress as much as possible by practicing midfulness, or awareness of the present moment. This is very important because stress is a toxic emotion and the concept behind fasting is to give your body rest and a chance to purify itself. You create stress for yourself when you start thinking about the thousands of things you need to do and all the problems that need to be solved. But keep in mind that you can only do one thing at a time in this present moment.

Let's now take a look at the most important guidelines on when to eat. Avoid junk foods or foods that are high in fat, processed and rich in "empty calories" as much as possible. This will safeguard your overall health. Make sure you eat fruits and vegetables, but don't be afraid to give yourself an extra once in a while (moderation is key).

Make sure you are aware of your calorie intake and treat it like it's on a budget. Try it as an experiment. Let's say you can eat up to 2,000 calories a day - that's it. This is your calorie budget for the day. You could spend it all at once, or you can spread it out throughout the day. You could eat just one thing that contains 2,000 calories, or you can choose a variety of different foods and follow a more balanced schedule.

It might be more difficult at first. Develop new habits gradually by decreasing your calorie intake and adding some physical activity. Give your body time to adjust to the new regimen and be patient with yourself. If you are hard on yourself, you will start to feel guilty and it is likely that you will give up entirely. The body has the ability to adapt.

3. Method 16: 8 benefits and side effects

The biggest advantage of the 16: 8 method is that your body will not go into "hunger mode" because you will eat and consume calories during your waking hours.

You can drink a lot of water as soon as you wake up; you can eat a plate of fresh fruit for breakfast at 11.00, then a salad and some protein for lunch; a small snack (like a handful of nuts for example) in the afternoon and a light dinner around 7pm.

During the 16-hour window your body will start using insulin and fat for energy. It doesn't matter if you are awake or asleep; your body will continue to burn calories for all of its different functions. These calories will come from stored fat. This is what makes 16: 8 intermittent fasting an effective weight loss program.

Intermittent fasting has various health benefits and this is probably one of the reasons why it is becoming more and more common.

One of the benefits of the intermittent fasting diet is that it reduces sudden hunger. Intermittent fasting regulates the production of leptin and ghrelin, which in turn reduces hunger and promotes satiety.

When produced in excess, the hunger hormone (ghrelin) prompts you to eat more. After a few days of intermittent fasting, ghrelin and leptin levels return to normal. Higher levels of leptin, on the other hand, curb hunger. These hormones play an important role in weight loss.

While most likely followed primarily for weight loss purposes, the intermittent fasting diet has a much broader list of benefits.

Following the trendy diets, instead of sticking to a healthy diet, is not only useless for the purposes of weight loss, but can even be harmful to the body. Too many changes in short periods of time can lead to various digestive problems, weight gain, and abdominal pain.

I suggest that you focus on feeling good and eating healthy without punishing yourself and without being too harsh and rigid. This means you may want to experiment with different methods and then decide what works for you. The reason why so many people are having success with the intermittent fasting program is that it is flexible (as we have seen you can decide between the various types of regimens) and quite simple.

Another important benefit of intermittent fasting is that it can help control blood sugar levels. This is essential because sugar spikes are the main cause of excess food intake and especially high-calorie food.

When you follow intermittent fasting appropriately for an extended period of time, you start to increase insulin resistance and lower blood glucose levels naturally.

While some people say you can eat whatever you want during the eating phase, being on some sort of weight loss program - or to improve health - requires you to be aware of what you eat and this leads to choices. healthier. This is another benefit of choosing the intermittent fasting diet.

Eating nutrient-rich foods, as opposed to junk food and what are called "empty calories", helps reduce weight, improve heart health, cholesterol and even bone structure.

While intermittent fasting can be an excellent tool to help you lose weight, it is still important to choose the food you eat carefully and to adopt healthier habits with respect to both nutrition and exercise.

In any case, keep in mind that there are some side effects to consider.

Now that we've seen the advantages, let's take a look at what are considered to be the disadvantages. Let's briefly review the side effects of the intermittent fasting diet.

One of the potential drawbacks of intermittent fasting is that the window of time you can eat is shorter. You may be used to eating smaller meals throughout the day instead of concentrating them over a set period of time.

One of the consequences, especially if you follow the warrior diet or other similar plan, is that you can feel too full and uncomfortable. This means that you can really struggle to stick to this diet because, during fasting you will suffer from hunger pangs, while you will feel annoyed by overeating during the period in which you are allowed to eat. Basically, you are never satisfied.

This is one of the reasons why I have suggested more than once not to force yourself and always pay attention to how you feel.

However, if you really want to try the more extreme methods, at least consume nutrient -rich foods as much as possible, so that you have adequate nutrition without feeling sick.

Another negative, and this happens with many diets, is that you find yourself constantly thinking about food and eating, basically becoming obsessed with the alternating phases of fasting and the period in which you can consume food.

This could also happen when you are with your friends or family. You may have to give up or put off a night out if your friends plan to coincide with your fasting phase.

Plus, just because something works for you doesn't mean it works for all of your friends, family, and colleagues too. So keep your eating plans and health goals to yourself without trying to convince everyone else to follow the same regimen as you. Even if you may have the best of intentions and really want to help them, your advice and suggestions will not be appreciated unless specifically requested.

Intermittent fasting doesn't have to become an obsession. It is a way to train yourself to listen to your body and understand it better. By this I mean that it causes you to pay attention to understand when he is really hungry, when he is satisfied, when he is feeling energetic and vital or when he is feeling tired and stressed.

This is a problem with many diets, they quickly become obsessive and often fail. The only way to make them work is to develop a healthy relationship with yourself and your body first and foremost. So treat food as fuel, not entertainment or a way to escape your emotional problems.

Some people wonder if it is possible to train while fasting and there are some contradictory theories on this subject. However, there are many studies that support the theory that training while fasting is possible and can even be beneficial. This is true for a short period of fasting (as in the 16: 8 method for example).

I suggest you pay attention to how you feel and start making changes little by little. Additionally, also remember to speak to your doctor before starting a diet or exercise program.

Knowing when to train during intermittent fasting is probably one of the most frequently asked questions. You can still do your regular workouts during intermittent fasting, you could just do a few lighter activities when you fast and choose more demanding activities during the eating window.

One of the drawbacks is reduced athletic ability, which may occur when fasting due to a lack of energy and strength. As suggested, to get around this problem you simply have to choose less intense activities during the fasting periods.

The intensity of your workouts can make a big difference. Suppose you like yoga and HIIT training (high intensity interval training), you could choose yoga during fasting and HIIT sessions during feeding phase.

If you decide to train while fasting, pay attention to cardio workouts. High-intensity cardio exercise, such as running or HIIT, can be a bit tiring for your body when you don't eat for an extended period of time. So just make sure you don't schedule your cardio workouts on days when you fast.

Many people who have followed the intermittent fasting diet suggest doing workouts just before starting the feeding phase. Of course, this can vary based on the type of training you do, how you feel, and how long you fast.

If you are following the 16: 8 method for example, you may want to do cardio after you enter the phase where you can eat, or at least you can consume a protein shake or a small healthy snack (like some nuts) before starting the strict routine.

Some people who have extremely intense training routines, such as crossfit, find they need a boost in protein and carbohydrates before a workout. If this is the case, you may need to do your workouts during the feeding phase and not the fasting phase.

Let's now look at the benefits of training during the intermittent fasting program. There are a number of reasons to do this, plan your workouts during the fasting period, as long as you don't feel sick or weak.

First of all, it helps your body get stronger and burn more fat. Exercising while fasting can also help with digestion. Many people find that eating just before or after a workout makes digestion more difficult, causing a variety of stomach problems.

Each person is different, each body is different and reacts in different ways to new nutrition and training programs. For this reason, it is really difficult to decide in advance which method would be best to follow.

As you can understand, the human body has amazing capabilities and adapts to extreme situations.

PART III
INTERMITTENT FASTING 16: 8
STEP-BY-STEP GUIDE

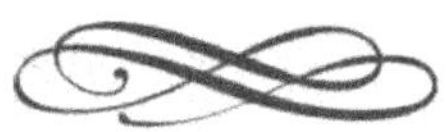

1. Method 16: 8: how to follow it

There has been a lot of research done for this version of the intermittent fasting diet. Research has shown this to be an effective way to help people lose weight, lower blood pressure, and reduce the risk of diabetes.

This method is much easier for most people to follow than other versions of the intermittent fasting diet that require 24 hours of fasting at a time if not up to 36.

Following the 16: 8 method, you fast for 16 hours, most of it at night while you sleep. There should be no calorie intake in this 16-hour window. You can drink plenty of water, especially in the morning when you wake up, and some unsweetened coffee or tea.

During the 8-hour window you can eat, make sure you are on a healthy and nutritious meal plan. It is not complicated and the benefits are worth trying.

Planning your meals is pretty straightforward if you choose the 16: 8

method. Previously, we suggested eating between 11am and 7pm. This tip is based on what is thought to be the simplest method, but it also depends on your daily schedule and activities.

That said, studies have shown that eating earlier in the evening is preferable to eating late and going to bed with a full stomach. So if, as in the example, you eat your last meal at 7pm and go to bed at 11pm, there is a lot of time between the meal and bedtime.

This doesn't mean you necessarily have to follow that method. It really depends on your lifestyle. If you want to choose to eat between 8.00 and 16.00 this is fine too. Just choose an 8-hour window in which you can eat and follow it with discipline, regardless of what others do (your family, your colleagues or friends ...).

Planning is something that will make it easier for you to stick to a new healthy diet. This means that you reduce the chances of ending up eating the first available thing.

If you exercise, you will need fuel to have enough energy to complete the exercise program. Fuel means nutrients, good energy for your body. The higher the percentage of wholesome and fresh foods in meals, the more likely you are to lose weight.

Whether you are following the 16: 8 method and fasting all night, or even if you are fasting two days a week, eat high calorie foods during non-fasting periods, or drink any type of beverage other than plain water, tea or coffee, it can still ruin your weight loss plans. This is because much of your calorie deficit is offset by an extremely high calorie intake during the feeding window and you won't be able to lose weight.

Many times people eat out of boredom, so keeping busy can be of great help. Watching TV makes you hungry, so try to minimize it. If you keep busy, you will be able to keep food cravings at bay and indeed enjoy the benefits of the intermittent fasting diet. You may want to plan fasting on busy days so you don't have time to obsess over food-related thoughts.

Some of the basic problems you may face during the first fasting period, such as the ones we just mentioned (overcoming boredom and a tendency to think about food; anger and sudden desires to eat), can be alleviated by drinking plenty of water and unsweetened coffee or tea in moderation. Green tea is also an excellent remedy for hunger pangs.

When it comes to drinks like coffee and tea, balance is always the key. Too much coffee can be harmful, a small amount can be helpful.

High levels of caffeine can cause problems related to the adrenal glands and consequently have a negative impact on long-term health, particularly when it comes to adrenal malfunction which can lead to thyroid problems, insomnia, excessive fat accumulation, low immunity and fatigue apart from a number of other serious problems.

Choose healthy fats (such as fish, extra virgin olive oil and nuts); proteins (poultry; lean meat; eggs); complex carbohydrates; fiber, vitamins and minerals are very useful, not only to normalize body weight, but to reduce hunger, glycemic peaks, fatigue and irritability.

If you are just getting started, and have never tried fasting before, you can experiment and see what works best for you. There are methods that vary in which fasting can go from one day to two days a week.

You can fast from lunch to lunch or from dinner to dinner and spread the fast over the two days where you can sleep the most. However, I would not suggest fasting for more than 24 hours.

Here are some extra tips you could follow when planning your schedule.

If you are adopting intermittent fasting to lose weight, you need to fit all your meals within the window.

Know your schedule, plan ahead. Intermittent fasting is primarily time based, and many people may tell you that it doesn't matter what food you eat during the you can eat phase. However, food is important. What you put into your body has an effect not only on how you look, but above all on how you feel.

This is an essential concept to understand any type of eating plan you intend to undertake. You could say: "but yes, a slice of cake or a dessert won't make a difference" but this is equivalent to focusing only on the aesthetic effect and will soon lead to giving up because the aesthetic results take time to be visible.

The question is, how do you feel? This is something you feel right away. How does a certain type of food make you feel? This is the question you need to ask yourself if you want to stick to your plans and achieve your goals.

That said, it is true that schedules are the concept behind the intermittent fasting diet and you need to stick to them in order for you to benefit from this diet.

The fasting interval can last from eight to 36 hours.

Let's now take a look at the most important guidelines on the fasting phase, especially if you decide to fast for more than 16 hours.

This phase is particularly useful for those who have to shed a lot of excess weight. As a good starting point, you could consider the idea of introducing some calories - in a reduced way - even during the fast and gradually reduce until following the actual fast in this phase.

The key is to make sure you maintain a stable power phase time. The times and the type of food you eat can be adjusted as you go. If you exercise, you will need more carbohydrates than fat for energy. We are obviously talking about healthy carbohydrates, not simple sugar. Complex carbohydrates such as whole grains, fruits and vegetables.

Likewise, on days when you are not exercising, it will be more important to take in fat. Healthy fats (think nuts, salmon, extra virgin olive oil, 100% natural nut butters like coconut or peanut butter).

Eat plenty of whole, unprocessed foods, and make sure you are consuming enough protein every day (eggs, lean meat, and fish).

It is important to pay attention to what you eat during the days you work out.

Many people who embark on intermittent fasting soon realize that their lives are marked by alternating phases of fasting and nutrition. In fact, this involves having to plan everything and always keep schedules under control. However, these drawbacks can be avoided with proper planning.

Keep in mind your routines and your needs, what are your daily schedules. What time do you wake up? What time is your lunch break at work? Do you prefer to eat when you wake up or do you prefer to go to sleep with a full stomach?

It is vital that you know your schedule and preferences. If you like to go to bed with a full stomach, you will probably need to schedule your eating window to start several hours after waking up. What if you're at work and hungry? Will you be able to take a break and have your first meal when the feeding phase begins?

All of these are considerations to keep in mind when choosing which intermittent fasting method you want to adopt and then plan your fast accordingly.

Now, just because the 16: 8 intermittent fasting method is easy to understand and simple to plan, that doesn't mean it's also easy to put into practice. Mainly because you have to be very disciplined in your meal times and also because you still have to be aware of what you eat and your calorie intake.

If you're just getting started with this method, give yourself some time to adjust to the new routine. In case you fail or fail to follow the regime the way you want it for some reason, don't think you've screwed it up or made a mistake. All of this will only make you feel miserable and will not bring good results.

Give yourself some time and if you happen to break the rules, just get back on track without making a fuss.

Here are the most common pitfalls you may want to avoid.

Indulge in too much junk food and sugary drinks and also snack late at night or after the 8-hour can eat phase.

If you're not losing weight or reaping any benefit from the 16: 8 intermittent fasting method, you may want to cut down on snacks and over-calorie foods.

Another trap is being afraid of hunger. This is because a mechanism is triggered by which you do nothing but think about food and consequently about hunger. If you follow the 16: 8 method, there is no reason to be afraid of being hungry because you will eat almost regularly. Plus, if you cut back on sugar (in all its many forms), eat a lot of fiber and protein, your body will adapt and you won't feel the need to eat all the time.

Focus on what you are doing moment by moment and keep in mind the final results you want to achieve. Remember that you can't get anything with nothing. Any goal you want to achieve requires effort.

If you are eating healthily and balanced during the eating phase but still not losing weight, it probably means that you are not getting enough exercise.

Exercise is essential not only for weight loss, but more generally, for your well-being. Just because you eat healthy and fast for 16 hours straight doesn't mean you'll automatically be toned and fit. You have to choose some kind of fun activity to move your body, keep it flexible and vital.

Many are tempted to want to use fasting as an excuse to move less, but don't fall into this trap. Especially if you have chosen the 16: 8 method.

You will realize that exercise actually releases more energy and as a result you will want to be even more active throughout the day in all the things you do. It will make you feel so much better.

If you follow the program I suggested (breakfast at 11.00 - lunch at 14.00 - small snack at 16.00 and dinner at 19.00) you could train for half an hour around noon or around 18.00. depending on your commitments. Just make sure you work out safely and not immediately after a meal, otherwise you may feel uncomfortable and have cramps.

If you're starting out, I suggest you avoid sharing your weight loss goals and diet plan with other people who might put you off. Sometimes sharing your plans with people who aren't supportive and supportive is like throwing water on a spark before it can ignite.

If you are planning a dinner with your friends or family, simply adjust your schedule for that day so that you can still fast for 16 hours. If other people you eat with decide to eat very high calorie and calorie-laden foods, you simply eat a lighter meal without having to explain or justify yourself.

If you feel uncomfortable, you can always say that you are not very hungry because maybe you ate too much during the previous meal or something else that comes to mind at that moment. The right thing to say will come if you relax and don't make a big deal out of it. I also learned that no one really tracks you except you, and that's probably always the case for everyone.

Another trick I've learned is to pretend I'm getting a call. Excuse yourself for a moment and when you get back to the table just say that you are finished and that you are no longer hungry. Again, don't make it seem like a big deal and no one will notice.

This is an important concept because even if you don't realize it on a more conscious level, the people you surround yourself with have a huge impact on your behavior.

These are the main tips you need to follow if you want to start a diet and more specifically if you have chosen the 16: 8 method. Try them to see if they are right for you. It just takes a little practice.

How to follow the 16: 8 method: additional helpful information

If there is one method of intermittent fasting that most people tend to try first, it is probably the 16: 8 protocol. This is mainly due to its simplicity.

I believe this protocol is particularly useful for beginners as you don't have to wait that long before eating.

Many people have a hard time following the intermittent fasting diet when they choose the method that takes 24 hours or more without eating. This is what is expected with the warrior method or the Eat-Stop-Eat method of intermittent fasting.

With the 16: 8 method, there are only a few hours in the morning and a few hours in the evening that you need to fast.

As your body gets used to the new protocol, you will be less hungry and above all you will feel hungry only when it is actually time to eat because the body will adapt to the new program.

If you like to go out at night, or if you are used to hanging out with friends, it might be best to start the fasting phase later, then skip breakfast and have a late lunch the next day. The 16 hours of fasting could be difficult but only for the first few days.

2. Intermittent diet: meal plan

7 Ideas for breakfast

- High protein smoothie

You can easily make a delicious and nutritious high-protein smoothie with avocado, almond milk (100% natural with no added sugar), fresh spinach leaves and protein powder.

With this smoothie you will feel full and satisfied thanks to the protein and healthy fats of avocado. Spinach will give you energy and a good supply of fiber.

Note: All green leafy vegetables are full of nutrients, be sure to consume plenty of them (spinach, kale, etc.)

If you prefer another type of plant-based milk, that's fine as long as you choose the healthiest option - the one that has fewer ingredients (that's why it's important to read the labels). You could buy spelled milk or oat milk etc.

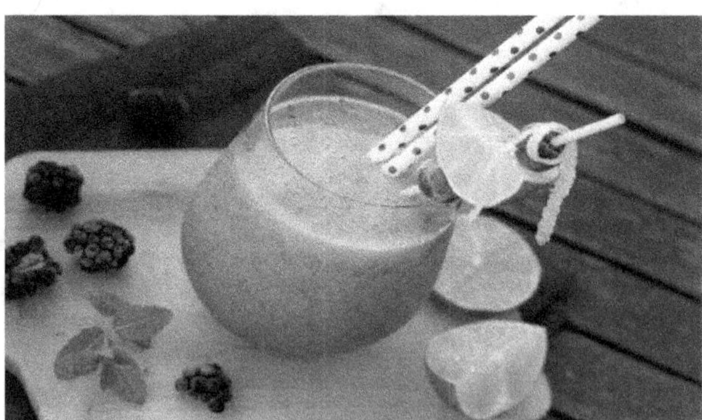

- Plate of fresh seasonal fruit

When you wake up, you have been fasting for a long time, which means that, especially at the beginning of your intermittent diet journey, your body craves carbohydrate-rich foods.

Bakery products, bread, croissants, focaccias etc ... If instead of succumbing to these temptations you prepare a plate of fresh fruit, you will do your body a great favor and it will reward you with a lot of energy.

Alternate according to your tastes, perhaps an apple and a banana with cinnamon on top. Strawberries, blueberries and grapes. A peach, some plums and apricots. The important thing is that it is fresh and without added sugars.

You could have a cup of unsweetened tea or plain coffee.

- *Vegetable omelette*

To make this omelette, you need to have pre-cooked vegetables, such as zucchini, spinach or carrots. Beat a couple of eggs, add a pinch of salt and black pepper, the vegetables and cook in a hot pan with a small piece of butter or a drizzle of oil.

Note: If you use butter, make sure it is of good quality. If you choose oil, make sure it is extra virgin olive oil.

Again, you could have a cup of unsweetened tea or plain coffee.

- *Natural low-fat yogurt (Greek type) with seeds and nuts*

When choosing what to eat, avoid the type of food that generates even more hunger. These are foods that are high in sugar, in all its forms. Simple carbohydrates, such as baked goods, are basically sugar.

Alternatively, you could try low-fat fresh Greek yogurt with berries and nuts. If you like, you can also add some cinnamon and a teaspoon of honey.

- *Oat flakes*

Buy fresh oats and cook it for a few minutes with a cup of hot water or half water and half your favorite vegetable milk. You can consume this oat mixture with fruit or nuts, cinnamon and honey.

- *Boiled egg and spinach*

Try two hard-boiled eggs at room temperature with a sprinkle of cinnamon and black pepper on top.

You can add fresh spinach leaves with natural raisins (sugar free). Or you can lightly brown the spinach in a pan with a drizzle of extra virgin olive oil or a little butter.

- *Whole grains*

A bowl of whole grains and your favorite plant-based milk. You can also add dried fruit to cereals for greater taste and above all a greater protein and nutritional intake.

Alternate and try these 7 breakfast ideas based on your tastes and what you have available. This type of breakfast will give you energy and nourish your body. You may still crave simple carbohydrates at first, but that's only a temporary thing. It's a habit. You can use these ideas for healthy snacks too, perhaps in smaller portions.

7 Ideas for lunch

The problem with lunch is that many people are usually not home during lunch. So if you are not used to preparing something to take with you, then you could consider it a problem ... I assure you that it is not that difficult, it is just a matter of habit and a little advance planning. Plus, the more simple you choose, the easier it will be to prepare a lunch to take with you when you go out.

Also, get freezer-safe containers that you can put in the fridge or microwave. This way you are equipped and will be able to eat your healthy meals.

- *Lettuce rolls*

You can easily make rolls with large lettuce leaves that you will fill with tuna and tomatoes. You can add fresh oregano or basil, a pinch of salt and pepper.

You can alternate lettuce with cabbage and you can substitute tuna with feta cheese or chicken strips.

- *Broccoli salad*

In a bowl, combine broccoli and thinly sliced peppers, black olives, and shallot. Prepare an emulsion with a little apple cider vinegar and extra virgin olive oil. Salt and pepper.

- *Lentil and cauliflower salad*

Steam the cauliflower florets for about 7 minutes, leave to cool and slice them. Cook the lentils in boiling water for about 35 minutes and let them cool. In a large bowl, mix the cauliflower and lentils, add the raisins and season with the Mediterranean emulsion which is very simple to make: whisk some fresh lemon juice and a drizzle of extra virgin olive oil. Add salt and pepper to taste.

- *Chicken and vegetable salad*

Lightly fry the vegetables in a pan with a drizzle of extra virgin olive oil, season with salt and pepper.

Grill the chicken breasts and season with some fresh Mediterranean herbs such as oregano or rosemary. You can eat this hot dish, with chicken and vegetables on the side, or you can let it all cool, then slice and mix them together in a bowl or container to take with you. I assure you that once you get used to this new method, you will be preparing these meals in less than 30 minutes.

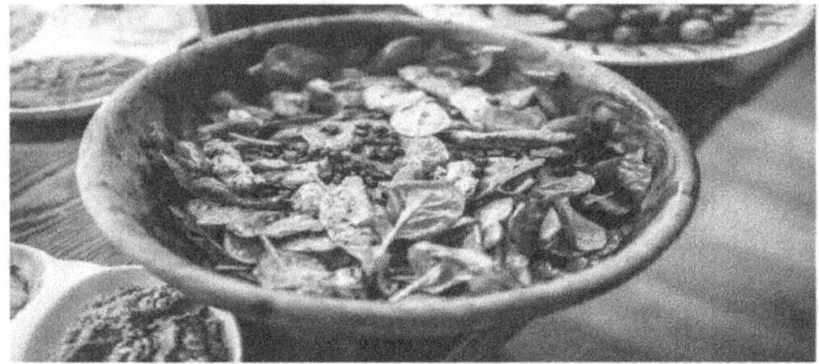

- *Beef strips with vegetables*

Cook the meat on a hot skillet and then slice it into thin strips. Cook a few green beans with extra virgin olive oil and half a cup of hot water until all the water has reduced and the beans are soft but not mushy.

Again, you can have this hot meal, with beef and vegetables on the side, or you can let it all cool then slice and mix it in a bowl or container to take with you.

- *Smoked salmon and rocket*

Place the smoked salmon on a tray (or container if you have to take it with you). Add thin avocado slices on top, pepper and fresh squeezed lemon juice. Serve the salmon with a side of rocket topped with the Mediterranean emulsion (beat the freshly squeezed lemon juice and a drizzle of extra virgin olive oil) and a little raisins.

- *Stuffed zucchini*

Steam the zucchini for about 3- 5 minutes then cut them in half and empty the contents carefully without breaking them to put the filling. If the courgettes are too long, it may be best to cut them in half first and then empty and fill them with meat.

Fill the zucchini with minced meat. Add salt and pepper, a drizzle of extra virgin olive oil and bake at 356 ° C for about 40 minutes.

You can alternate between these meals and you could even use them as dinner ideas depending on your tastes and what you have on hand.

7 Ideas for dinner

These ideas could be useful for you and your family to eat wholesome foods and enjoy a healthy lifestyle. They are easy to make with simple ingredients and they taste really good.

Did you know that once you start eating healthy and keep doing it for a while, junk food will smell, look and taste disgusting to you? This is exactly what happens. It's like people who smoke and then quit smoking, after a while they can't tolerate the smell of cigarettes anymore.

- *Mediterranean-style stuffed eggs*

Soak white beans (cannellini beans) in hot water the night before making this recipe. (They need about 6/8 hours of soaking).

Cook the beans in boiling water for 40/50 minutes.

You need some hard-boiled eggs, let them cool, then divide them in half and empty them.

For the filling, you will need to create a mousse with the firm yolk, cannellini beans, tuna, fresh parsley, salt, pepper, a tablespoon of extra virgin olive oil and a little water. Use a hand blender to make the mousse.

2. Vegetable omelette

Cook the spinach in a pan with a little butter for a few minutes, season with salt. Beat two eggs with a pinch of salt and pepper. Add the eggs to the spinach. Cook on both sides for about 3/4 minutes.

You can replace the spinach with your favorite vegetables like green beans, broccoli, zucchini or kale.

3. Brown rice and vegetables

You can eat a little rice every now and then preferably brown rice of the best quality possible. Cook according to package directions and season with stir-fried vegetables, grilled chicken, or turkey.

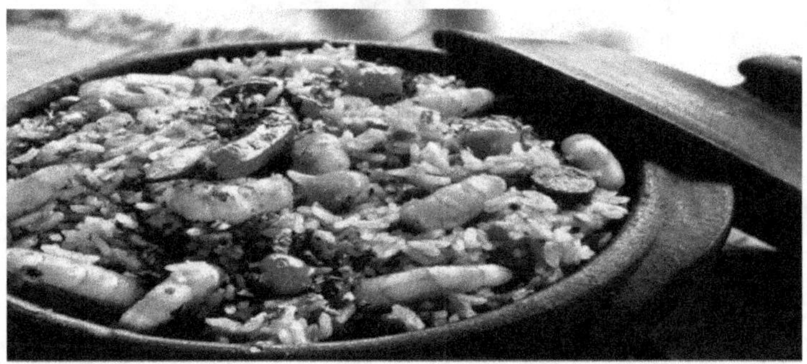

4. Grilled salmon with vegetables

Add sesame seeds on top of the salmon and cook it on the grill or in a hot pan. If you can, buy fresh, wild salmon. Serve with a side of chopped cabbage, carrots and radishes dressed with the Mediterranean emulsion (beat the juice of a fresh squeezed lemon and a drizzle of extra virgin olive oil).

5. Chicken with salad and dried fruit

This is a delicious salad that you can make with chicken, thinly sliced celery; fresh seedless grapes cut in half and walnuts. Season with salt and pepper; low-fat Greek yogurt and a drizzle of organic honey.

6. Sweet potatoes and chicken

Boil the sweet potatoes in hot water, mash them and season with butter; salt, pepper and cinnamon. Cook the chicken legs in a pan with garlic, extra virgin olive oil, curry, prunes (about 3 for each chicken leg) and bay leaves. Lightly brown the thighs on each side, then add about two cups of water. Cover with a lid and cook until all the water has reduced (usually about 50 minutes for three legs).

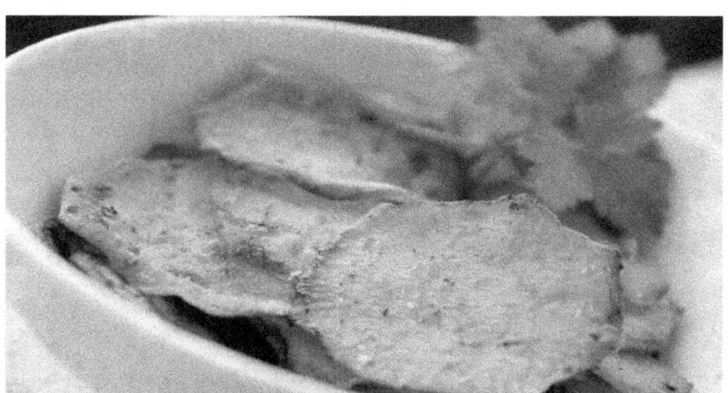

7. Greek Salad

The Greek salad is really fresh and healthy. You can make it very simply with rocket, feta cheese, thinly sliced onions, black olives, thinly sliced tomatoes, a thinly sliced apple and raisins. Season with the Mediterranean emulsion (beat the juice of a fresh lemon and a drizzle of extra virgin olive oil), salt, pepper and fresh oregano.

You can consume this salad with a slice of good quality wholemeal bread (fresh not packaged) and a drizzle of extra virgin olive oil.

As you can see, the recipes I've suggested contain protein, lots of vegetables, some complex carbohydrates, and fewer simple carbohydrates.

There is no real secret to being healthy, just know the macronutrients, how foods affect the body and follow common sense.

INTERMITTENT FASTING:
EASY STRATEGY
(EXTRA INFORMATION AND TIPS)

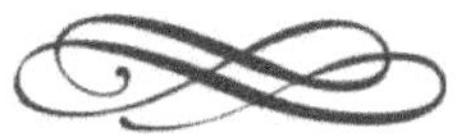

Make sure you stay hydrated. Whether you are an expert on fasting or if you've never tried it before, I can't stress enough the importance of staying hydrated.

When your body detoxifies itself, on fasting days, and starts releasing some of the toxins it has accumulated from years of junk food, it will make a lot less effort if you drink enough plain water.

As we have seen, there are various protocols that can be followed in the context of intermittent fasting and each has different rules. Some people choose to fast for 12-16 hours. Others plan a 72-hour fast.

While it is true that there are several protocols of intermittent fasting, there are basically two main approaches. The first alternates between days in which it is possible to eat and days of fasting. The second variant is what you will see in intermittent fasting diets such as the 5: 2 diet. This requires you to eat regularly for five days and fast for two days.

Much of the information I have provided on the intermittent fasting diet works well with all methods. Some people prefer the first approach for long-term results in terms of weight loss, ease of use, and the likelihood of being able to stick to the program.

Focus on eating healthy and staying active. This is the only effective key. No secrets and no mysteries.

If you have trouble fasting, remember that one of the secrets is getting distracted. Try yoga or Pilates, go out for a walk, drink herbal tea, or get more sleep. If you stick to this plan long enough, your eating habits will improve significantly.

CONCLUSION

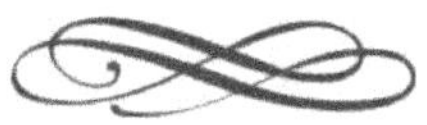

The body is a complex and sophisticated system that needs adequate   nutrients to function efficiently. These days we are faced with a constant onslaught of tempting junk foods and non-nutritious and addicting snacks.

Food has become a kind of entertainment.

At the same time, we lead more sedentary lives, made easier by technology and other devices to do things for us. As a result, our physical activity level dropped to alarming levels.

Shopping is now also done mostly online. We don't even have to leave the house anymore, not even wanting for food shopping. We could virtually do everything by just sitting somewhere with an internet connection.

The result is an increase in obesity and laziness and a loss in recognition of the benefits of genuine ingredients and a much simpler life.

Many, if not most, health problems could be avoided with proper nutrition and a healthier lifestyle. Spending time outdoors instead of looking at the screen all day would definitely help.

Our ancestors, as we have seen, had very different habits and obesity was not a real problem then. They were used to being more active and eating less. Their body had both strength and stamina to withstand the worst conditions, including prolonged hunger (fasting).

The intermittent fasting diet - if followed correctly - is one of the ways we can enjoy the benefits of a healthy life.

In this Guide we have highlighted a number of ways to overcome all your fears related to the possibility of adapting to fasting. But remember that it's all about effort, progress and consistency. And this is true regardless of the goal you want to achieve.

Also, we have delved into the 16: 8 method, but you can still explore all the other methods as well. One of the bencfits of the intermittent fasting diet is that you can really tailor it to you, based on your needs.

Fasting is one of the simplest ways that will allow you to freely choose from a number of healthy food options. You can select any of the suggested recipes and start today too.

Also remember to combine fasting with an exercise routine, even as simple as running. Exercising will increase your metabolic rate, especially fat oxidation. Completing your diet routine with exercise will allow you to reach your goals in a considerably shorter time.

Also, while you fast and check your calorie intake, resist the temptation to consume junk food. It might be difficult at parties and with friends, but try to plan your schedule so you can stick to your plans without giving up on your social life.

If you find that things are getting too stressful, make some changes to your plan, don't be too rigid. If you stop for any reason, don't blame yourself, start over. The point is to increase the quality of your life and feel better inside and out.

As we said at the beginning of this book, keep the goal in mind and remind yourself of the benefits of intermittent fasting.

With the knowledge and information provided and a positive approach, there's no reason why you won't be able to achieve your goals, whether it's weight loss, muscle gain, or overall health improvement.

Finally, please note that this Guide is for informational purposes only. Always consult your doctor before embarking on a diet or exercise program.